AI Sleep, Stress & Nervous System Reset

How Artificial Intelligence Restores Calm, Energy & Healing

By Joe Correa

Published by Live Stronger Faster

This book is for educational and informational purposes only. The author and publisher are not engaged in rendering legal, financial, or other professional advice. Readers should consult a qualified professional before making any financial decisions.

First Edition

Table of Contents

Introduction

Sleep, stress, and the nervous system form the hidden operating system of the human brain. Long before conscious thought, productivity, memory, or emotional regulation come into play, the nervous system decides whether the body is in a state of safety or survival. Modern life has quietly disrupted this foundational system. Chronic stress, artificial light, digital overload, irregular sleep cycles, emotional pressure, and constant stimulation have pushed millions of nervous systems into a permanent state of dysregulation. Burnout is no longer an exception; it has become the baseline. This book explores how artificial intelligence is emerging as one of the most powerful tools ever developed to reset, regulate, and restore the nervous system at scale.

For decades, sleep disorders, anxiety, chronic fatigue, and stress-related illness were treated as separate problems. Insomnia was handled by sleep medicine, anxiety by psychology, burnout by lifestyle advice, and nervous system disorders by neurology. What modern neuroscience has revealed is that these are not separate systems at all. They are expressions of a single network: the autonomic nervous system, the circadian rhythm, and the brain's stress response loops. When this network is dysregulated, everything else begins to fail. Artificial intelligence is uniquely positioned to intervene here because it can observe patterns the human brain cannot, respond in real time, and adapt interventions continuously rather than relying on static protocols.

AI does not replace rest, therapy, or healing. Instead, it enhances the brain's ability to recognize when it is safe to relax, recover, and repair itself. Through sleep-stage monitoring, biometric feedback, circadian rhythm optimization, stress pattern detection, and adaptive behavioral guidance, AI is becoming a digital nervous system assistant—one that learns how an individual body responds to stress and sleep deprivation and then guides it back toward equilibrium. This book examines how that process works, why it is effective, and what it means for human health in an age of constant stimulation.

The nervous system evolved to respond to short bursts of danger followed by long periods of recovery. Modern environments have inverted that equation. The brain now experiences low-grade stress continuously, without the clear resolution signals that once allowed it to return to baseline. Artificial intelligence excels at identifying these unresolved stress loops. By analyzing sleep data, heart rate variability, breathing patterns, cortisol rhythms, and behavioral signals, AI systems can detect when the nervous system is stuck in fight-or-flight or freeze states—even when the individual feels "normal." This invisible awareness is one of AI's greatest contributions to brain healing.

Sleep is the primary gateway through which the nervous system resets itself. During deep sleep, the brain clears metabolic waste, consolidates memory, repairs neural tissue, and recalibrates emotional responses. Yet millions of people never reach consistent deep sleep. AI-driven sleep systems now monitor sleep architecture in real time, learning how different stimuli, behaviors, and environments affect each sleep stage. Unlike traditional sleep advice, these systems personalize interventions, adjusting light exposure, sound, breathing cues, temperature, and timing to gently guide the brain into restorative states. This book explores how those technologies work and why personalization is essential for nervous system healing.

Stress is not simply a mental experience; it is a physiological state encoded into neural circuits. Chronic stress reshapes the brain, reinforcing hypervigilance, emotional reactivity, and cognitive fatigue. AI tools trained on stress biomarkers can detect early warning signs long before burnout becomes visible. By intervening early—through adaptive breathing protocols, micro-recovery prompts, sleep optimization, and nervous system retraining—AI helps prevent long-term damage rather than merely managing symptoms. This proactive model represents a fundamental shift from reactive healthcare to predictive brain wellness.

One of the most powerful insights explored in this book is that calm is not the absence of stress but the presence of regulation. The nervous system must be taught how to downshift. AI systems can act as patient, consistent trainers, reinforcing regulation patterns through repetition, timing, and feedback. Over time, this training rewires neural pathways, strengthening parasympathetic activation and reducing stress sensitivity. What once required years of trial-and-error therapy can now be guided with precision, supported by data rather than guesswork.

Burnout is often misunderstood as exhaustion alone, but it is fundamentally a nervous system injury. The brain loses its ability to switch off. Sleep becomes shallow, focus deteriorates, emotional resilience collapses, and motivation fades. AI-powered recovery systems are beginning to address burnout at its neurological root by rebuilding the brain's capacity for rest. This book explores how AI identifies burnout patterns, differentiates them from depression or anxiety, and designs recovery pathways that restore energy without forcing productivity prematurely. The integration of AI into nervous system regulation also raises important ethical and philosophical questions. What happens when machines help decide when humans should rest? How much data should be collected about sleep, stress, and emotional states? How do we ensure these tools empower rather than control? This book does not shy away from these questions. Instead, it frames AI as a support system—one that works best when aligned with human autonomy, consent, and biological wisdom.

This volume is not about futuristic speculation. The technologies discussed here already exist and are being used by clinicians, researchers, and individuals seeking deeper recovery. From AI-driven sleep platforms to adaptive stress-response training and nervous system biofeedback, these tools represent a quiet revolution in health. They shift the focus from pushing the brain harder to teaching it how to rest better, heal faster, and perform sustainably.

As part of the larger **AI Neuroplasticity & Brain Healing** series, this book serves a crucial role. Where previous volumes explored learning, emotional regulation, memory, and behavior change, this book addresses the foundation that makes all of those possible. Without sleep, calm, and nervous system balance, neuroplasticity becomes fragile. With them, healing accelerates. AI does not force the brain to change; it creates the conditions under which change becomes natural again. By the end of this book, readers will understand how artificial intelligence interacts with the nervous system, why sleep is the most powerful neurological intervention available, and how stress can be retrained rather than endured. More importantly, they will see how the future of recovery is shifting away from willpower and toward intelligent systems that help the brain remember how to rest, reset, and renew itself. This is not the end of human resilience—it is its intelligent evolution.

Chapter 1

The Nervous System: The Master Control Center of Sleep, Stress, and Recovery

The human nervous system is not simply a background biological process; it is the command center that determines how the brain experiences reality. Every sensation of calm or panic, clarity or exhaustion, focus or overwhelm originates from how the nervous system interprets the environment. Long before conscious thought intervenes, the nervous system has already decided whether the body is safe, threatened, energized, or depleted. Understanding this system is essential to understanding sleep, stress, and recovery—and it is the foundation upon which artificial intelligence now operates as a powerful regulatory tool.

At its core, the nervous system is divided into two primary branches: the sympathetic and parasympathetic systems. The sympathetic system prepares the body for action, heightening alertness, increasing heart rate, elevating cortisol, and sharpening attention. The parasympathetic system does the opposite, slowing the heart, lowering blood pressure, promoting digestion, deep sleep, tissue repair, and emotional regulation. In a healthy organism, these systems oscillate fluidly throughout the day. In modern life, however, this balance is increasingly rare.

Chronic stress has forced millions of nervous systems into a near-constant sympathetic state. Emails, notifications, deadlines, financial pressure, artificial lighting, disrupted sleep schedules, and emotional overload all signal the brain that vigilance is required. The nervous system responds accordingly, maintaining elevated arousal long after the original stimulus has passed. Over time, this state becomes normalized. The individual no longer feels "stressed" in the traditional sense, yet the body remains locked in a defensive posture that quietly erodes sleep quality, immune function, emotional resilience, and cognitive performance.

Sleep is where the nervous system is meant to reset itself. During deep sleep, parasympathetic dominance allows the brain to repair neural tissue, clear metabolic waste, regulate emotional memory, and recalibrate stress thresholds. When the nervous system cannot downshift, sleep becomes fragmented, shallow, and inefficient. The brain may remain active, replaying stress loops even while the body lies still. This creates a feedback loop in which poor sleep increases stress sensitivity, and heightened stress further degrades sleep. Traditional approaches to sleep and stress management often fail because they treat symptoms rather than regulation.

Advice such as "relax more," "sleep earlier," or "reduce stress" assumes that the nervous system can voluntarily shift states. In reality, dysregulated nervous systems cannot simply be commanded into calm. They must be retrained. This is where artificial intelligence introduces a fundamentally different approach.

AI excels at pattern recognition across complex, dynamic systems. When applied to nervous system regulation, AI does not rely on subjective reporting alone. It analyzes objective signals such as heart rate variability, breathing rhythms, sleep architecture, movement patterns, temperature fluctuations, and behavioral timing. Over time, it learns how an individual nervous system responds to stress, rest, stimulation, and recovery. This learning allows AI systems to intervene with precision rather than generalization.

For example, instead of recommending a generic bedtime, AI can identify when an individual's parasympathetic activity naturally increases and guide sleep timing accordingly. Instead of offering static breathing exercises, AI can adapt breath pacing in real time based on physiological response. Instead of waiting for burnout to appear, AI can detect early warning signals—subtle declines in recovery efficiency that precede fatigue, anxiety, or insomnia by weeks or months. The nervous system responds best to consistency and predictability. AI provides both. Unlike human coaches or therapists, AI systems do not fatigue, forget, or lose patience. They reinforce regulation gently and continuously, using micro-adjustments rather than drastic interventions. Over time, these small corrections compound, reshaping neural pathways and restoring the brain's ability to self-regulate.

Another critical advantage of AI-guided nervous system regulation is its ability to personalize recovery. No two nervous systems are identical. Genetics, trauma history, lifestyle, and environment all shape stress responses. What calms one person may activate another. AI learns these differences, avoiding the one-size-fits-all trap that undermines many wellness programs. This personalization accelerates recovery while reducing frustration and resistance.

Importantly, AI does not replace the body's natural intelligence. It augments it. The nervous system already knows how to regulate itself; it has simply lost the conditions required to do so consistently. AI helps recreate those conditions by aligning external cues—light, sound, timing, pacing—with internal biological rhythms. In this sense, AI acts as a translator between modern environments and ancient neural architecture.

As this chapter establishes, the nervous system is the gateway through which sleep, stress, and healing pass. Without regulation, no amount of productivity optimization or cognitive enhancement can succeed sustainably. With regulation restored, the brain regains its capacity for resilience, focus, and renewal. The chapters that follow will explore how AI applies these principles in practice. But first, it is essential to see how these abstract mechanisms unfold in a real human life.

The Quiet Collapse

Daniel did not think of himself as burned out. He was still functioning. He woke up early, answered emails, attended meetings, exercised sporadically, and met deadlines. From the outside, nothing appeared broken. Yet each night, sleep slipped further away. He lay in bed exhausted but alert, his mind replaying conversations, planning tomorrow, revisiting yesterday. When sleep came, it was light and easily disturbed. He woke up tired, but he told himself that was normal.

Over months, Daniel's body adapted to this state. Coffee replaced rest. Evenings blurred into screens. Weekends no longer refreshed him. He felt strangely disconnected from calm, as if relaxation were something he remembered rather than experienced. Doctors found nothing alarming. Blood work was normal. Stress management advice sounded reasonable but impossible to implement. His nervous system had forgotten how to stand down. One evening, after another restless night, Daniel noticed something unsettling: his heart raced during moments that should have been neutral. A delayed email, a minor decision, a trivial inconvenience triggered disproportionate tension. His body reacted as though danger were everywhere. This was not anxiety in the dramatic sense; it was vigilance without relief. He was trapped in readiness.

At the suggestion of a colleague, Daniel tried an AI-guided sleep and stress monitoring system. At first, he was skeptical. He assumed it would simply tell him what he already knew—that he needed more sleep and less stress. Instead, the system showed him patterns he had never noticed. His heart rate variability remained suppressed even during rest. His nervous system failed to enter parasympathetic dominance at night. His deepest sleep phases were brief and inconsistent.

The system did not instruct Daniel to "relax." It adjusted his environment subtly. Lights dimmed earlier. Sound frequencies shifted to encourage slower breathing. Notifications paused at precise times based on his stress response rather than a fixed schedule. Breathing cues adapted in real time, slowing only when his body followed rather than forcing compliance.

At first, the changes felt insignificant. But within weeks, Daniel noticed something new: moments of spontaneous calm. His body exhaled without effort. Sleep deepened in fragments, then in stretches. Mornings became clearer. He did not feel euphoric—he felt normal again. The most surprising change was emotional. Situations that once triggered tension now passed without hijacking his body. His nervous system began to trust safety again. This trust compounded. As sleep improved, stress sensitivity declined. As stress declined, sleep stabilized. The feedback loop reversed.

Months later, Daniel realized that recovery had not come from working harder or thinking differently. It had come from regulation. AI had not healed him directly; it had taught his nervous system how to remember itself. What once felt like a quiet collapse had become a quiet restoration—one breath, one night, one signal at a time.

Chapter 2

How Artificial Intelligence Detects, Interprets, and Rebalances Stress

Stress is not a single event but a continuous signal-processing problem inside the brain. Every moment, the nervous system evaluates incoming information and decides whether to mobilize energy or conserve it. When this process functions well, stress rises and falls naturally. When it fails, stress becomes chronic, invisible, and destructive. Artificial intelligence is uniquely capable of intervening in this failure because it can observe stress as a system rather than a feeling.

The human brain experiences stress long before the conscious mind labels it. Changes in breathing rhythm, heart rate variability, muscle tension, sleep timing, attention patterns, and emotional reactivity occur automatically. Most people become aware of stress only after it has accumulated enough momentum to feel overwhelming. By that point, the nervous system has already adapted to a heightened baseline. AI operates upstream of awareness, identifying stress signatures in real time and responding before conscious distress emerges.

Traditional stress management relies heavily on self-reporting. Individuals are asked how stressed they feel, how well they slept, or how anxious they are. These methods are limited by perception, memory, and normalization. A chronically stressed person often reports feeling “fine” because their nervous system has recalibrated what fine means. AI bypasses this limitation by focusing on physiology rather than perception. It does not ask how stressed someone feels; it measures how the body behaves.

Through continuous data collection, AI systems identify patterns that indicate nervous system overload. Reduced heart rate variability signals diminished parasympathetic activity. Irregular breathing patterns suggest persistent sympathetic activation. Fragmented sleep architecture reveals an inability to downshift. Micro-behaviors—such as increased nighttime movement, delayed sleep onset, or early awakening—provide additional context. Individually, these signals may seem insignificant. Together, they form a stress fingerprint unique to each person.

Once this fingerprint is established, AI can differentiate between acute stress and chronic dysregulation. Acute stress is adaptive and temporary. Chronic stress is persistent and maladaptive. This distinction is critical. Treating adaptive stress as pathology can reduce resilience, while ignoring chronic stress leads to burnout and illness. AI’s strength lies in recognizing when the nervous system has lost flexibility rather than simply reacting strongly. Interpretation is only the first step. The true power of AI lies in how it responds. Instead of issuing generalized advice, AI systems deploy targeted interventions aligned with the nervous system's current state. If the system detects hyperarousal, it may introduce slower breathing cues, auditory rhythms, or environmental adjustments that encourage parasympathetic engagement. If it detects under-arousal masked by fatigue, it may adjust light exposure, timing, or activity prompts to restore balance rather than induce further suppression.

Importantly, AI does not attempt to eliminate stress. Stress is necessary for learning, adaptation, and survival. The goal is regulation, not avoidance. AI-guided regulation trains the nervous system to move fluidly between states rather than remaining stuck. This flexibility is the hallmark of a healthy nervous system and the foundation of resilience.

One of the most overlooked aspects of stress is its cumulative nature. Stress does not reset at the end of the day. It accumulates when recovery is incomplete. AI tracks recovery efficiency rather than just stress exposure. Two individuals may experience identical stressors, yet recover at vastly different rates. AI identifies this discrepancy and adjusts interventions accordingly, focusing on improving recovery capacity rather than reducing external demands alone. Over time, AI-guided stress regulation reshapes neural circuits. Repeated exposure to well-timed regulation signals strengthens pathways associated with calm, safety, and restoration. The nervous system learns through experience, not instruction. AI provides consistent experiences of regulation, allowing the brain to internalize new patterns. What begins as external guidance becomes internalized self-regulation.

This process also reduces cognitive load. Many stress interventions require conscious effort, which paradoxically adds strain to an already overloaded system. AI reduces the need for decision-making by automating regulation cues. The nervous system responds directly to sensory input without requiring analysis or willpower. This efficiency makes AI particularly effective for individuals who are exhausted, burned out, or overwhelmed.

Ethically, AI-driven stress regulation must prioritize transparency and autonomy. The goal is not to optimize humans for productivity but to restore balance. Well-designed systems empower users by revealing patterns and offering choices rather than enforcing compliance. This alignment is essential for trust and long-term effectiveness.

As this chapter demonstrates, AI does not merely detect stress; it interprets context, adapts interventions, and retrains the nervous system over time. Stress becomes a signal to be managed intelligently rather than endured blindly. To understand how this transformation unfolds in daily life, we turn now to a story that illustrates stress detection and rebalancing from the inside.

The Signal Beneath the Noise

Maria had learned to ignore stress. As a project manager, she believed pressure was part of the job. Deadlines, messages, shifting priorities—it all blended into a constant hum. She told herself she was handling it well. She still met expectations. She still exercised occasionally. She still slept, or at least she lay in bed long enough to call it sleep.

What Maria did not notice was how her body had changed. Her breathing was shallow even at rest. Her jaw remained clenched without awareness. She woke up tired, not from lack of hours, but from lack of depth. Weekends no longer reset her. She carried tension into moments that should have been light.

When her company offered access to an AI-based stress and recovery platform, Maria enrolled out of curiosity. She assumed it would confirm what she already knew—that she was busy but functional. Instead, the system revealed a pattern she could not argue with. Her stress markers never fully resolved. Even during rest, her nervous system remained activated. She was not experiencing stress spikes; she was living inside a sustained stress signal.

At first, the system made small adjustments. Breathing cues appeared during moments of subtle tension rather than obvious distress. Soundscapes shifted when her heart rate variability dropped. Notifications paused not according to schedules, but according to physiological strain. Maria barely noticed these changes consciously, yet her body responded.

Within days, something unfamiliar happened. She caught herself exhaling deeply without effort. Her shoulders dropped spontaneously. These moments were brief but undeniable. The system continued adapting, learning when her nervous system resisted and when it followed. It did not force calm; it waited for cooperation.

As weeks passed, Maria noticed a deeper shift. Stressful events still occurred, but they no longer lingered. Her body returned to baseline more quickly. Sleep deepened. She woke up feeling restored rather than merely awake. The background hum softened.

The most profound change came unexpectedly. One evening, after a long day, Maria realized she felt present. Not distracted, not vigilant—present. Her nervous system was no longer scanning for the next demand. It was resting in safety. Maria understood then that stress had not been her enemy. Dysregulation had been. AI had not removed pressure from her life; it had taught her nervous system how to recover. The signal beneath the noise had finally been heard—and answered.

Chapter 3

Sleep as a Neurological Reset: How AI Restores the Brain's Natural Recovery Cycles

Sleep is not rest in the passive sense; it is an active neurological reconstruction process. Every night, the brain enters a complex sequence of stages designed to restore cognitive clarity, emotional balance, immune strength, and nervous system regulation. When these stages are disrupted, recovery becomes incomplete, and stress accumulates invisibly. Artificial intelligence is transforming sleep from a fragile, unpredictable event into a guided neurological reset by understanding sleep as a system rather than a habit.

The brain cycles through distinct phases during sleep, each serving a unique function. Light sleep initiates disengagement from the external world. Deep sleep repairs tissue, clears metabolic waste, and stabilizes the nervous system. REM sleep integrates memory, processes emotion, and recalibrates stress responses. These stages must occur in a precise rhythm. Disruption at any point weakens the entire recovery process. AI's role is to preserve this rhythm by identifying when and why it breaks down. Modern sleep problems rarely stem from a lack of opportunity to sleep. They arise from an inability to transition into restorative states. The nervous system often remains partially alert, monitoring for threats that no longer exist. Artificial light, late-night stimulation, irregular schedules, emotional stress, and unresolved cognitive loops all interfere with the brain's ability to surrender control. AI detects these barriers not as abstract causes but as physiological signals expressed through delayed sleep onset, fragmented cycles, shallow deep sleep, and premature awakening.

Unlike traditional sleep tracking, which focuses on duration alone, AI analyzes sleep architecture. It examines how long each stage lasts, how smoothly transitions occur, and how consistently cycles repeat. This depth of analysis reveals whether sleep is truly restorative or merely prolonged unconsciousness. Two individuals may sleep eight hours; one wakes restored, the other exhausted. AI identifies the difference and responds accordingly.

One of AI's most powerful contributions to sleep recovery is timing optimization. The brain follows circadian rhythms governed by light exposure, temperature, hormonal cycles, and behavioral cues. When sleep timing conflicts with these rhythms, even long sleep becomes inefficient. AI learns an individual's biological timing and adjusts sleep windows dynamically rather than enforcing fixed schedules. This alignment reduces friction between the nervous system and the environment.

AI also addresses hyperarousal, one of the most common barriers to deep sleep. Hyperarousal occurs when the sympathetic nervous system remains active at night, preventing full parasympathetic dominance. AI-guided interventions target this state subtly, using breath pacing, sound modulation, temperature adjustments, and cognitive unloading techniques. These interventions work not by suppressing alertness forcefully, but by signaling safety consistently until the nervous system responds.

Another overlooked factor in sleep recovery is micro-awakenings. These brief interruptions often go unnoticed consciously but fragment sleep cycles significantly. AI detects patterns that lead to micro-awakenings, such as environmental noise, physiological discomfort, or stress-related neural activity. By addressing these triggers, AI improves sleep continuity, allowing deeper stages to unfold uninterrupted.

Over time, AI-guided sleep recovery produces compounding benefits. As sleep deepens, stress sensitivity declines. As stress declines, sleep stabilizes further. Emotional regulation improves. Cognitive clarity sharpens. The nervous system regains confidence in rest. This virtuous cycle contrasts sharply with the downward spiral many individuals experience when poor sleep and chronic stress reinforce each other.

Importantly, AI does not aim to maximize sleep metrics artificially. The goal is not perfect scores but functional recovery. Well-designed systems prioritize adaptability over optimization, recognizing that sleep needs fluctuate with life demands. By responding to context rather than enforcing rigid ideals, AI supports sustainable recovery rather than performance obsession.

Sleep is the most powerful natural intervention for nervous system healing. AI enhances its effectiveness by removing friction, restoring rhythm, and reinforcing regulation. As this chapter demonstrates, sleep is not something to be forced or hacked; it is something to be protected, guided, and trusted. The following story illustrates how restoring sleep architecture through AI can transform not just nights, but waking life itself.

The Longest Night Ends

Ethan had forgotten what deep sleep felt like. He slept every night, yet each morning felt like a continuation of the day before. His body was heavy, his thoughts slow, his emotions muted. He told himself this was adulthood—that fatigue was normal, that rest was optional. Night after night, Ethan lay in bed while his mind replayed unfinished conversations and imagined future problems. He did not feel anxious exactly; he felt alert. His nervous system refused to disengage. Even when sleep arrived, it was fragile. Dreams were vivid but unsatisfying. He woke often without knowing why.

When Ethan began using an AI-guided sleep recovery system, the first insight unsettled him. He was not sleeping poorly because he lacked discipline. His sleep architecture was fractured. Deep sleep occurred in short bursts, frequently interrupted. REM cycles were shallow and delayed. His nervous system never fully trusted the night.

The system did not demand earlier bedtimes or strict routines. Instead, it adjusted Ethan's environment gradually. Light exposure shifted earlier in the evening. Sound cues softened during moments of physiological alertness. Breathing rhythms slowed when his body resisted, then paused when it complied. The system waited for cooperation rather than imposing control.

The first night Ethan slept deeply startled him. He woke up disoriented—not from exhaustion, but from unfamiliar restoration. His body felt heavier in a comforting way. His mind was quieter. He realized he had not dreamed intensely; he had rested.

Over the following weeks, sleep became something Ethan looked forward to rather than endured. Micro-awakenings diminished. Mornings grew clearer. Emotional reactions softened. The constant undercurrent of fatigue faded.

One evening, sitting quietly, Ethan noticed something extraordinary: he felt calm without effort. His nervous system had relearned how to shut down. Sleep had become a place of safety again.

Ethan understood then that sleep had never abandoned him. His nervous system had simply forgotten how to enter it. AI had not replaced his body's wisdom; it had reminded it. The longest night had ended—not with force, but with guidance.

Chapter 4

Burnout, Fatigue, and Nervous System Collapse: How AI Rebuilds Energy from the Inside Out

Burnout is not a lack of motivation, discipline, or resilience. It is a neurological shutdown caused by prolonged nervous system overload without adequate recovery. When the nervous system is pushed beyond its regulatory capacity for too long, it does not simply become tired—it adapts by conserving energy at all costs. This adaptation manifests as fatigue, emotional numbness, cognitive fog, sleep disruption, and loss of drive. Artificial intelligence is uniquely positioned to address burnout because it recognizes exhaustion not as weakness, but as a signal of systemic failure in regulation.

The nervous system is designed to prioritize survival over performance. When stress remains unresolved, the brain begins to downregulate energy output to prevent further damage. This protective response is often misinterpreted as laziness or depression. In reality, it is a strategic withdrawal. Burnout represents the nervous system's final attempt to force rest when conscious behavior refuses to allow it. AI reframes burnout as data—information about where regulation has failed and recovery must begin. Traditional burnout interventions often focus on surface-level changes: time off, reduced workload, motivation strategies, or mindset shifts. While helpful temporarily, these approaches rarely address the underlying dysregulation that caused burnout in the first place. Without restoring nervous system balance, individuals return from rest only to relapse. AI intervenes at a deeper level by identifying the physiological markers of burnout long before collapse occurs and guiding recovery with precision.

Burnout is characterized by specific patterns: persistently low heart rate variability, disrupted circadian rhythms, blunted emotional responses, fragmented sleep, and reduced stress adaptability. AI systems trained on these patterns can differentiate burnout from depression, anxiety, or acute stress. This distinction matters. Treating burnout as depression may further suppress nervous system activity. Treating it as stress may push an already depleted system harder. AI enables targeted recovery rather than misdirected intervention.

Energy restoration begins with safety. The burned-out nervous system does not respond to stimulation; it responds to reassurance. AI-guided recovery systems reduce unnecessary demands on the nervous system by automating regulation cues, simplifying decision-making, and pacing reactivation carefully. Instead of forcing productivity, AI helps the nervous system relearn that rest is allowed and recovery is possible.

One of AI's most critical roles in burnout recovery is pacing. Burned-out individuals often oscillate between overexertion and collapse. AI smooths this cycle by identifying optimal activity thresholds and preventing overextension. By monitoring recovery signals continuously, AI adjusts expectations in real time, protecting fragile gains and preventing setbacks.

Sleep plays a central role in burnout recovery, but sleep alone is insufficient if the nervous system remains hypervigilant or suppressed. AI integrates sleep optimization with daytime regulation, ensuring that recovery is reinforced across the full 24-hour cycle. This holistic approach allows energy to rebuild gradually rather than spike temporarily.

As recovery progresses, AI supports gentle reactivation of engagement and motivation. This process is subtle. The nervous system must be invited back into activity, not coerced. AI recognizes early signs of readiness—improved recovery efficiency, stabilized sleep cycles, increased emotional range—and responds by expanding capacity incrementally. This avoids the boom-and-bust pattern common in burnout recovery.

Importantly, AI reframes energy as a renewable resource rather than a finite one. Burnout teaches the nervous system to hoard energy defensively. AI-guided regulation demonstrates that energy can be spent and restored safely. Over time, this retraining rebuilds trust between the brain and the body.

Burnout recovery is not about returning to the old normal. It is about establishing a new equilibrium that prioritizes regulation, rhythm, and sustainability. AI supports this transition by making invisible processes visible and guiding behavior without adding cognitive load. As this chapter illustrates, burnout is not the end of capacity—it is the beginning of a necessary neurological reset.

The story that follows shows how burnout unfolds quietly, how recovery begins subtly, and how AI-guided nervous system restoration can return vitality without force or urgency.

The Weight of Empty Days

Lena used to measure her life in output. Projects completed. Goals met. Problems solved. She thrived on motion. Then, slowly, motion stopped rewarding her. Tasks that once energized her began to feel heavy. Decisions felt exhausting. Even rest felt ineffective.

At first, Lena blamed herself. She tried to push through, assuming she had lost discipline. She took short breaks, planned vacations, read productivity books. Nothing worked.

Her sleep became shallow. Her emotions flattened. She no longer felt stressed—she felt empty.

What Lena did not realize was that her nervous system had shut down to protect her. Years of unresolved pressure had taught her brain that effort led to depletion. So it withdrew.

When Lena began using an AI-guided recovery system, the initial feedback was sobering. Her recovery metrics were severely compromised. Even rest failed to restore her nervous system. She was not tired; she was depleted.

The system did not urge action. It reduced stimulation. It slowed her days. It adjusted sleep timing and sensory input. It removed friction rather than adding tasks. At first, Lena felt restless, even guilty. Doing less felt wrong.

Then something shifted. One afternoon, she noticed a flicker of interest in a conversation. Another day, she laughed unexpectedly. These moments were brief but real. The system recognized them and responded by allowing slightly more engagement.

Weeks passed. Energy returned slowly, unevenly. The system protected Lena from overdoing it, gently pulling her back when recovery lagged. For the first time, she trusted the pace. Months later, Lena realized she felt alive again—not driven, not pressured, but present. She understood then that burnout had not taken her strength. It had forced her to rebuild it correctly.

AI had not healed her by pushing harder. It had healed her by listening—to signals she had ignored for years. The weight of empty days lifted, replaced by something quieter and stronger: sustainable energy.

Chapter 5

Rewiring Safety, Calm, and Focus: How AI Trains the Nervous System for Long-Term Stability

A regulated nervous system is not defined by the absence of stress, but by the presence of safety. Safety is a neurological state in which the brain determines that survival is not immediately threatened and resources can be allocated toward learning, focus, creativity, and repair. When safety is absent, the nervous system prioritizes vigilance over clarity. Artificial intelligence plays a transformative role in restoring this sense of safety by retraining the brain through repetition, predictability, and precision.

The nervous system learns through experience, not instruction. Telling someone to feel calm does nothing if the nervous system has learned that calm is unsafe. Many individuals live with nervous systems shaped by prolonged stress, trauma, instability, or unpredictability. In such systems, calm itself can feel unfamiliar or even threatening. AI recognizes this paradox and approaches regulation gradually, allowing the nervous system to relearn safety without force. At the neurological level, safety is associated with consistent parasympathetic activation, stable breathing rhythms, coherent heart rate variability patterns, and reduced threat scanning. These signals must be experienced repeatedly to be trusted. AI excels at delivering these experiences consistently. By monitoring physiological responses in real time, AI can introduce regulation cues only when the nervous system is receptive, reinforcing positive patterns rather than triggering resistance.

Focus emerges naturally from safety. A nervous system that is not scanning for danger can allocate attention efficiently. In contrast, a dysregulated system experiences distractibility, mental fatigue, and fragmented concentration. AI-guided regulation improves focus not by demanding productivity, but by stabilizing the conditions under which attention becomes effortless. This distinction is critical. Focus is an outcome of regulation, not a skill to be forced.

One of AI's greatest strengths is its ability to remove uncertainty. The nervous system is highly sensitive to unpredictability. Unclear schedules, erratic demands, and inconsistent feedback keep the brain in a heightened state of alert. AI introduces rhythm and predictability through adaptive routines that align with biological needs rather than arbitrary rules. Over time, this consistency retrains the nervous system to expect safety instead of disruption. AI also supports emotional regulation by stabilizing physiological baselines. Emotions are not purely psychological; they are embodied states influenced by nervous system activity. When the nervous system is regulated, emotional responses become proportional and transient. When it is dysregulated, emotions linger, intensify, or flatten. AI-guided interventions normalize emotional processing by addressing the physiological substrate beneath emotional experience.

Importantly, long-term stability requires more than acute regulation. The nervous system must internalize new patterns until they become automatic. AI facilitates this internalization by providing continuous feedback loops. As regulation improves, AI gradually reduces external guidance, allowing the nervous system to assume control. This transition from dependence to autonomy is essential for sustainable change.

Focus, calm, and safety are mutually reinforcing. As calm increases, focus sharpens. As focus stabilizes, stress sensitivity decreases. AI supports this upward spiral by maintaining alignment between internal state and external demands. When demands exceed capacity, AI signals the need for adjustment. When capacity expands, AI allows engagement to increase. This dynamic calibration prevents regression while promoting growth. Over time, AI-guided nervous system training reshapes identity. Individuals no longer see themselves as anxious, unfocused, or overwhelmed. They experience these states as temporary fluctuations rather than fixed traits. This shift reduces self-judgment and reinforces resilience. Regulation becomes the default, not the exception.

As this chapter illustrates, long-term nervous system stability is not achieved through willpower or suppression. It is built through repeated experiences of safety, delivered with precision and respect for biological limits. Artificial intelligence does not replace human agency; it creates the conditions under which agency can flourish. The following story illustrates how this retraining unfolds quietly, reshaping focus, calm, and confidence from the inside out.

Learning What Calm Feels Like

Aaron had always been productive, but never peaceful. His mind moved quickly, jumping between tasks, ideas, and worries. Focus came in bursts, followed by exhaustion. He told himself this was just how he was wired. Calm felt foreign, almost suspicious.

Even during moments of rest, Aaron's body remained alert. His breathing was shallow. His thoughts raced. Silence felt uncomfortable. He filled it with noise, work, or stimulation. He did not realize that his nervous system had learned to associate stillness with danger. When Aaron began using an

AI-guided nervous system training platform, the first challenge surprised him. The system did not push him to meditate or concentrate harder. Instead, it focused on creating brief moments of safety. Slower breathing. Predictable rhythms. Gentle cues that faded when his body resisted.

At first, these moments felt awkward. Aaron noticed a strange urge to escape them. The system detected this response and adjusted, shortening sessions and reducing intensity. It waited for his nervous system to consent.

Gradually, something shifted. Aaron began to recognize calm as a physical sensation rather than an abstract idea. His shoulders dropped. His breath deepened. Focus emerged without effort. These moments grew longer, then more frequent.

Weeks passed. Aaron's productivity improved, but not through force. Tasks that once drained him now felt manageable. Distractions lost their grip. He noticed emotions passing through him instead of sticking. Calm no longer felt dangerous; it felt familiar.

One afternoon, sitting quietly without a screen, Aaron realized he felt safe. Not bored. Not restless. Safe. His nervous system had learned something new.

AI had not taught him how to focus. It had taught his nervous system that it was allowed to rest. From that rest, focus arose naturally. Calm was no longer something he chased—it was something he carried.

Chapter 6

Integration, Resilience, and Long-Term Nervous System Maintenance in an AI-Augmented World

True nervous system recovery is not a single achievement but a maintained state of adaptability. A healthy nervous system is not one that remains calm at all times, but one that can move fluidly between activation and rest without becoming stuck. The goal of AI-guided nervous system training is not permanent relaxation, but durable resilience—the capacity to respond, recover, and reengage without cumulative damage. This chapter explores how artificial intelligence supports long-term regulation by integrating recovery into daily life rather than isolating it as a separate practice.

Once safety, sleep, energy, and focus have been restored, the nervous system enters a phase of consolidation. During this phase, new regulatory patterns must be reinforced until they become automatic. Without reinforcement, the nervous system may revert to old survival strategies under pressure. AI plays a critical role during consolidation by maintaining subtle guidance while gradually reducing dependence. This tapering process ensures that regulation is internalized rather than outsourced.

Long-term nervous system health depends on rhythm. Biological systems thrive on predictable cycles of effort and recovery. Modern environments disrupt these rhythms by demanding constant availability, rapid response, and sustained attention. AI counters this disruption by reintroducing rhythm through adaptive scheduling, recovery prompts, and capacity tracking. These systems do not impose rigid routines; they respond dynamically to fluctuations in stress, sleep quality, and emotional load.

Resilience emerges when the nervous system trusts that recovery will follow effort. In dysregulated systems, effort feels dangerous because recovery has historically failed. AI rebuilds this trust by ensuring that recovery is consistent and sufficient. Over time, the nervous system becomes willing to engage fully again, knowing it will not be abandoned afterward. This trust transforms how individuals approach work, relationships, and challenges.

Maintenance also involves recognizing early warning signals. A regulated nervous system does not collapse suddenly; it signals strain long before breakdown occurs. AI excels at detecting these early shifts—subtle changes in recovery efficiency, sleep architecture, or emotional reactivity—and responding before they escalate. This preventive capacity distinguishes AI-guided regulation from reactive self-care.

Another essential aspect of long-term stability is identity integration. Individuals who have lived in chronic stress often identify with vigilance, productivity, or endurance. Recovery can feel disorienting, even threatening, to this identity. AI supports identity transition by normalizing regulation as strength rather than weakness. As calm and focus become consistent, individuals begin to redefine competence around sustainability rather than sacrifice.

AI also facilitates boundary formation. Boundaries are not merely psychological constructs; they are physiological limits. A regulated nervous system recognizes when engagement exceeds capacity. AI reinforces this recognition by translating physiological signals into actionable guidance. Over time, individuals learn to respect these signals independently, strengthening autonomy rather than dependence.

Importantly, long-term nervous system maintenance does not mean avoiding stress. Growth requires challenge. AI supports adaptive stress by distinguishing between constructive strain and destructive overload. It allows the nervous system to stretch safely, recover efficiently, and expand capacity gradually. This balance fosters growth without relapse. As artificial intelligence becomes more integrated into daily life, ethical alignment remains essential. AI must serve human well-being rather than optimization for output alone. Systems designed for nervous system health prioritize consent, transparency, and flexibility. They empower users to understand their bodies rather than surrender control. This alignment ensures that AI enhances human agency rather than eroding it.

Ultimately, AI-guided nervous system maintenance represents a shift in how health is understood. Recovery is no longer episodic. Regulation is no longer reactive. Stability is no longer fragile. Instead, the nervous system becomes a responsive, resilient foundation upon which learning, creativity, longevity, and emotional depth can flourish. This integration prepares the brain not only for rest, but for the expanded possibilities explored in the books that follow.

The final story illustrates what it means to live with a regulated nervous system—not as a peak experience, but as a quiet, sustainable way of being.

The Return of Capacity

Noah remembered when effort felt expensive. Every decision drained him. Every commitment carried an invisible cost.

Even after recovery began, he feared relapse. He waited for the exhaustion to return, certain it would.

At first, Noah relied heavily on AI guidance. It reminded him to slow down, to rest, to disengage. It protected him from overcommitment. Gradually, those reminders became less frequent. His body responded before prompts appeared. His nervous system had learned.

Months passed. Stressful events still happened—deadlines, conflicts, uncertainty—but they no longer lingered. Noah noticed something subtle yet profound: recovery followed effort naturally. He no longer braced for collapse after busy days. Sleep restored him. Calm returned on its own.

One afternoon, Noah declined an opportunity without guilt. He felt his limits clearly and respected them. Another day, he pushed himself slightly and recovered fully. These moments built trust. His nervous system no longer saw life as a threat.

The AI system faded into the background. It was still there, watching quietly, intervening only when necessary. Noah realized he no longer needed constant guidance. Regulation had become internal.

Years earlier, Noah had believed resilience meant endurance. Now he understood it meant responsiveness. His nervous system was no longer something he fought or ignored—it was something he partnered with. Walking home one evening, Noah felt present. Not hyper-aware. Not numb. Present. His body moved with ease. His mind was clear. Calm was no longer a goal. It was the ground he stood on.

AI had not changed who Noah was. It had given him back the capacity he had lost—and taught him how to protect it. The nervous system reset was complete, not as an ending, but as a foundation for everything that came next.

Chapter 7

The Regulated Brain as the Foundation for Human–AI Integration

Before the human brain can safely interface with advanced neurotechnology, it must first be regulated. Regulation is the prerequisite for integration. A nervous system that is chronically dysregulated cannot distinguish enhancement from overload, assistance from intrusion, or signal from noise. Artificial intelligence, when used first as a stabilizing force rather than an augmenting one, prepares the brain for deeper interaction with technology by restoring clarity, boundaries, and trust at the neurological level.

Human–AI interaction already occurs constantly, often unconsciously. Notifications, algorithms, recommendation engines, and digital feedback loops shape attention, emotion, and behavior. When the nervous system is dysregulated, these interactions amplify stress and fragmentation. When the nervous system is regulated, the same technologies become supportive tools rather than sources of overwhelm. This distinction is critical. The future of AI and neurotechnology depends not on more powerful machines, but on healthier human nervous systems capable of engaging them selectively and intentionally. A regulated brain maintains a clear sense of agency. Agency is not a philosophical abstraction; it is a physiological state. When the nervous system feels safe, the brain can evaluate information without urgency. It can pause, reflect, and choose. Dysregulation collapses this capacity, replacing choice with reaction. AI-guided nervous system training restores agency by reducing baseline threat perception, allowing higher cognitive functions to operate consistently.

As AI systems become more immersive—through wearables, adaptive environments, and eventually direct neural interfaces—the importance of regulation increases exponentially. A brain that cannot disengage will be vulnerable to dependency, over-stimulation, or cognitive fatigue. A regulated brain, by contrast, can enter and exit AI-mediated states fluidly, preserving autonomy while benefiting from augmentation.

Integration requires coherence across systems. Sleep, stress response, emotional regulation, focus, and energy must operate in synchrony. AI establishes this coherence by aligning internal rhythms with external inputs. Over time, the brain learns to recognize coherence as its default state. This recognition becomes a protective mechanism, allowing the nervous system to detect misalignment quickly and correct course. One of the most significant risks of advanced neurotechnology is cognitive overload. Information delivered faster than the nervous system can integrate it creates fragmentation rather than enhancement. AI-guided regulation trains the brain to process information efficiently, prioritizing depth over volume. This capacity will be essential as interfaces evolve from passive tools into interactive systems that respond directly to neural signals.

Another critical factor is emotional integrity. Emotions guide decision-making, empathy, and moral reasoning. Dysregulated nervous systems distort emotional signals, leading to impulsivity, numbness, or reactivity. Regulation restores emotional clarity, ensuring that AI-augmented cognition remains grounded in human values rather than purely computational efficiency.

The regulated nervous system also establishes healthy boundaries with technology. Boundaries are not imposed cognitively; they are felt physiologically. AI-guided regulation helps individuals sense when engagement becomes excessive and disengage without guilt or fear. This capacity protects long-term mental health and preserves the human role in decision-making.

As this book has demonstrated, AI's first and most important role is not enhancement, but restoration. By repairing sleep, recalibrating stress, rebuilding energy, and stabilizing focus, AI prepares the nervous system for the next phase of human–technology evolution. Without this foundation, neurotechnology risks amplifying dysfunction. With it, integration becomes empowering rather than invasive.

Chapter 7 closes this volume by reframing regulation as readiness. The regulated brain is not passive or diminished; it is prepared. Prepared to learn faster, adapt deeper, and engage technology without losing itself. The story that follows illustrates what it feels like to live in this state of readiness—where calm, clarity, and agency coexist with intelligence, ambition, and growth.

Standing at the Threshold

Sophia used to feel overwhelmed by technology. Her days were filled with screens, updates, and constant input. Even tools designed to help her felt demanding. She blamed herself for not keeping up, unaware that her nervous system was already overloaded before each interaction began.

After months of AI-guided nervous system regulation, something changed. Technology no longer felt intrusive. Notifications lost their urgency. Information arrived without pressure. Sophia noticed she could engage deeply, then disengage completely. This was new. When she began experimenting with more advanced AI tools—adaptive learning systems, immersive environments, intelligent assistants—she felt something unexpected: control. Not dominance, but partnership. Her nervous system remained calm as complexity increased. She could sense when to continue and when to stop.

Sophia realized that the difference was not the technology. It was her nervous system. She no longer met information from a place of threat. She met it from stability. Her brain absorbed what was useful and released the rest.

One evening, reflecting on her progress, Sophia understood that recovery had not made her less ambitious. It had made her more precise. Her energy was focused. Her emotions were clear. Her decisions felt aligned.

Standing at this threshold, Sophia did not fear the future of AI. She felt ready for it. Her nervous system was no longer something she managed—it was something she trusted. And in that trust, she recognized the true promise of human–AI integration: not replacement, not control, but collaboration.

The reset was complete. The foundation was laid. What came next would build upon regulation, not replace it.

Chapter 8

Awareness, Presence, and Conscious Regulation: How AI Helps the Brain Observe Itself Without Fear

The final stage of nervous system regulation is not control, but awareness. Once the nervous system is stable, rested, and resilient, the brain gains the capacity to observe its own internal states without being overwhelmed by them. This capacity—often described as presence, mindfulness, or consciousness—is not mystical. It is neurological. Artificial intelligence, when applied correctly, does not replace this awareness but helps reestablish the biological conditions under which it naturally emerges.

In dysregulated nervous systems, awareness feels dangerous. Attention directed inward amplifies discomfort, anxiety, or threat signals. This is why many people struggle with mindfulness or meditation despite sincere effort. The nervous system interprets stillness as exposure. AI-guided regulation resolves this problem by restoring safety first. Only when safety is established can awareness unfold without triggering defense.

Awareness is the nervous system's ability to track sensation, emotion, and thought without immediate reaction. This ability depends on a stable autonomic baseline, balanced neurotransmitter activity, and coherent neural oscillations. AI supports these conditions by maintaining regulation beneath awareness, allowing observation to occur without effort. In this way, awareness becomes a byproduct of stability rather than a task to be performed.

Once awareness emerges, it becomes a powerful regulatory force. The brain begins to recognize stress patterns as they arise, rather than after they escalate. Emotions are felt fully but briefly. Thoughts are noticed rather than believed automatically. This meta-awareness reduces cognitive fusion and emotional reactivity, strengthening resilience without suppression.

AI enhances this process by providing gentle mirrors. Rather than instructing the user to focus inward, AI reflects patterns externally—changes in breath, heart rhythm, sleep depth, or stress recovery—allowing the brain to correlate internal experience with physiological state. Over time, the nervous system learns to sense these shifts independently. Awareness becomes embodied rather than conceptual.

Presence also alters the experience of time. Dysregulated

nervous systems feel rushed or frozen. Regulated systems experience time as spacious and flexible. AI-guided rhythm restoration supports this shift by aligning internal pacing with external demands. As time pressure dissolves, awareness deepens naturally.

Importantly, awareness does not eliminate discomfort. It changes the relationship to it. A regulated nervous system can experience discomfort without interpreting it as danger. AI reinforces this distinction by preventing escalation while allowing sensation to be felt. This capacity is foundational for emotional intelligence, creativity, and ethical decision-making.

As awareness stabilizes, individuals report a sense of coherence—a feeling that thoughts, emotions, and actions are aligned. This coherence is measurable neurologically as synchronized neural activity across regions involved in attention, emotion, and executive function. AI supports coherence by reducing noise and reinforcing integration across systems.

Awareness also protects against overidentification with technology. A brain capable of observing its own state can engage AI without surrendering autonomy. It recognizes when assistance is helpful and when disengagement is necessary. This discernment is critical as AI becomes more immersive and persuasive. At this stage, AI's role becomes increasingly subtle. Guidance fades into the background. The nervous system assumes responsibility for regulation. Awareness sustains itself through experience rather than instruction. AI remains present as a safety net rather than a driver.

Chapter 8 represents the culmination of nervous system reset—not as an endpoint, but as an opening. Awareness is the platform upon which deeper meditation, expanded consciousness, and intentional human–AI collaboration are built. The story that follows illustrates how awareness returns quietly, transforming perception without fanfare.

Watching the Mind Without Running

Elena used to avoid silence. In quiet moments, her thoughts grew loud, her body tense. Stillness felt like exposure. She filled every gap with sound, movement, or distraction, unaware that her nervous system equated awareness with danger.

After months of AI-guided regulation, something softened. Elena noticed pauses appearing naturally. Not forced, not planned—just moments where nothing demanded her attention. At first, these moments felt unfamiliar. Then they felt welcome.

One evening, sitting alone without her phone, Elena realized she was observing her thoughts instead of chasing them. They rose and fell like weather. Her body remained calm. There was no urgency to fix or escape anything.

The AI system had not instructed her to meditate. It had simply ensured her nervous system was safe enough to notice itself. Breath slowed. Heart rhythm stabilized. Awareness arrived on its own.

Over time, Elena began recognizing early stress signals—a tightening chest, shallow breath—before they intensified. She responded gently, without judgment. Regulation became intuitive. Presence became familiar.

The most profound shift was emotional. Elena felt emotions fully, but they no longer overwhelmed her. Sadness passed. Joy lingered. Anger dissolved without damage. Awareness created space.

One afternoon, walking through a crowded street, Elena felt grounded. Noise did not intrude. Movement did not exhaust her. She was present within complexity, not protected from it.

Elena understood then that awareness was not something she had to achieve. It was something her nervous system had always known how to do. AI had not given her consciousness—it had removed the barriers that hid it.

Watching the mind no longer felt like running toward danger. It felt like coming home.

Chapter 9

Longevity Begins with Regulation: How AI Protects the Brain from Aging, Decline, and Cognitive Erosion

Longevity is not determined solely by genetics or the passage of time; it is shaped continuously by how the nervous system manages stress, recovery, and energy over decades. The brain ages fastest under conditions of chronic dysregulation. Sleep deprivation, unresolved stress, inflammation, and persistent sympathetic activation accelerate neural wear, impair repair mechanisms, and erode cognitive reserve. Artificial intelligence alters this trajectory by protecting the nervous system at its most fundamental level, slowing decline not through force, but through regulation.

Neurodegeneration does not begin suddenly. It emerges gradually as the cumulative cost of incomplete recovery. Each night of fragmented sleep, each prolonged stress response, and each period of emotional suppression leaves a trace. Over time, these traces accumulate into measurable changes in brain structure, neurotransmitter balance, and network connectivity. AI-guided regulation interrupts this accumulation by ensuring that recovery becomes consistent rather than occasional. Sleep is the primary neuroprotective mechanism available to the human brain. During deep sleep, the brain clears metabolic waste, reduces inflammation, and consolidates neural pathways. Disrupted sleep impairs these processes, accelerating cognitive aging. AI improves sleep not merely by increasing duration, but by preserving sleep architecture over the long term. This preservation protects memory, attention, and emotional processing well into later life.

Stress is another powerful accelerator of brain aging. Chronic cortisol exposure damages hippocampal neurons, impairs neurogenesis, and weakens synaptic plasticity. AI mitigates this damage by reducing baseline stress activation and shortening recovery time after stress exposure. The nervous system learns to return to equilibrium efficiently, minimizing cumulative harm.

Inflammation links stress, sleep, and aging into a single pathway. Dysregulated nervous systems promote systemic inflammation, which in turn affects brain health. AI-guided regulation reduces inflammatory signaling indirectly by restoring autonomic balance. This systemic effect highlights why longevity cannot be addressed through isolated interventions alone. The nervous system must be stabilized as a whole. Cognitive reserve—the brain's ability to compensate for age-related changes—depends on regulation. A regulated brain learns more efficiently, adapts more flexibly, and recovers more completely. AI supports cognitive reserve by maintaining optimal conditions for plasticity across the lifespan. Rather than pushing performance, it preserves capacity.

As individuals age, nervous system resilience becomes increasingly important. Recovery slows naturally with time. AI adapts to these changes by adjusting expectations and pacing. What once required brief rest may require longer recovery later in life. AI respects this shift, preventing frustration and injury by aligning activity with biological reality.

Importantly, longevity is not about avoiding challenge. Cognitive engagement and learning remain essential for brain health. AI supports healthy challenge by ensuring that engagement occurs within a regulated nervous system. This balance allows growth without exhaustion, stimulation without damage.

Neuroprotection also involves emotional health. Chronic emotional suppression accelerates cognitive decline. AI-guided awareness and regulation allow emotions to be processed rather than stored somatically. This emotional fluidity protects neural networks involved in memory and decision-making.

As this chapter demonstrates, AI's role in longevity is subtle but profound. It does not promise immortality or radical enhancement. It preserves what already exists. By stabilizing the nervous system, AI slows the erosion of brain health, extending not just lifespan, but healthspan—the years in which cognition, presence, and agency remain intact.

The story that follows illustrates what longevity feels like from the inside—not as endless youth, but as sustained clarity, adaptability, and vitality across time.

The Years That Did Not Steal Him

Marcus used to believe aging was something that happened all at once. One day, you woke up slower, foggier, less sharp. He watched older colleagues decline quietly and assumed the same fate awaited him.

In his forties, stress dominated Marcus's life. Sleep was inconsistent. Workdays were long. Recovery felt optional. He told himself he would rest later.

When Marcus began using AI-guided nervous system regulation, he expected short-term relief. Instead, something deeper occurred. His sleep stabilized. Stress responses softened. Recovery became reliable.

Years passed. Marcus noticed something unusual. While peers complained of forgetfulness and fatigue, he felt clear. Not invincible—just intact. His mind adapted. His energy returned after exertion. He still felt emotions deeply, but they moved through him rather than lodging in his body.

As Marcus entered his sixties, he realized that time had not taken what he expected. He still learned quickly. Conversations energized him. Quiet moments felt rich rather than empty. His nervous system responded to challenge without panic.

AI had not reversed aging. It had slowed damage. It had protected recovery. It had preserved rhythm. Marcus understood that longevity was not about resisting time—it was about cooperating with it.

Sitting one evening, watching the light fade, Marcus felt present. Not nostalgic. Not fearful. Present. His nervous system was calm. His mind was clear. The years had passed, but they had not stolen him.

AI had not extended his life unnaturally. It had allowed him to live it fully, one regulated day at a time.

Chapter 10

From Regulation to Evolution: The Nervous System Reset as the Gateway to Human Potential

The nervous system reset is not a wellness trend or a temporary intervention; it is a structural upgrade to how humans live, learn, and evolve in a technologically accelerated world. Throughout this book, sleep, stress, recovery, focus, awareness, and longevity have been examined not as isolated functions, but as expressions of a single system. Chapter 10 brings these threads together to show why nervous system regulation is the gateway to sustainable human potential—and why artificial intelligence, when aligned correctly, becomes a catalyst rather than a crutch.

Human potential has always been limited not by intelligence, but by regulation. Brilliant minds collapse under chronic stress. Creative insight disappears under exhaustion. Emotional depth is blunted by survival mode. The nervous system decides how much of the brain's capacity is available at any moment. When dysregulated, it narrows possibility. When regulated, it expands it. AI's most transformative contribution is not increasing intelligence, but restoring access to it.

Regulation changes how the brain interprets challenge. In a dysregulated state, challenge is threat. In a regulated state, challenge is information. This shift alters learning speed, decision quality, emotional resilience, and ethical reasoning. AI supports this transformation by ensuring that stress responses resolve fully and consistently, preventing the accumulation that erodes capacity over time.

The nervous system reset also redefines productivity. Instead of extracting output from exhausted systems, productivity becomes an emergent property of clarity and energy. AI-guided regulation replaces the boom-and-bust cycle with sustainable engagement. Over time, individuals discover that doing less with more presence produces better results than doing more under strain.

One of the most profound outcomes of regulation is coherence—the alignment of thought, emotion, behavior, and physiology. Coherence is measurable neurologically and perceptible subjectively. It feels like integrity. AI supports coherence by reducing noise, synchronizing rhythms, and reinforcing recovery. This coherence becomes the foundation for advanced learning, creativity, leadership, and collaboration.

As AI systems grow more capable, the regulated nervous system becomes a form of protection. It guards against manipulation, overload, and dependency. A regulated brain can pause, evaluate, and choose. It can partner with AI without surrendering agency. This capacity will define the difference between empowerment and erosion in the future of human–AI interaction.

Importantly, regulation is not about minimizing intensity or ambition. It is about expanding tolerance. A regulated nervous system can experience intensity without fragmentation, ambition without burnout, and complexity without confusion. AI enables this expansion by continuously calibrating load and recovery, ensuring that growth does not outpace repair.

The nervous system reset also carries moral implications. Ethical judgment requires emotional clarity and cognitive flexibility. Chronic dysregulation narrows empathy and accelerates reactive decision-making. Regulation restores the neural conditions necessary for compassion, foresight, and responsibility. In this way, nervous system health becomes a prerequisite not just for performance, but for wisdom.

This book has demonstrated that AI is most powerful when it works beneath consciousness rather than competing with it. By stabilizing the nervous system, AI allows awareness, creativity, and insight to emerge naturally. The future of intelligence is not artificial replacing human—it is artificial supporting human regulation so that human intelligence can operate fully.

Chapter 10 reframes the nervous system reset as evolution rather than recovery. It is the transition from surviving modern life to participating in it consciously. From reacting to choosing. From enduring to engaging. AI does not dictate this evolution—it enables it by restoring the biological foundation upon which it depends.

The story that follows is not about extraordinary achievement. It is about ordinary life lived with extraordinary coherence. It illustrates what it means to move forward after the reset—not into perfection, but into possibility.

The Day Nothing Needed Fixing

On a quiet morning, Julian noticed something unusual: nothing felt urgent. Not in a careless way, but in a grounded one. His body felt awake without tension. His mind was clear without effort. He was not trying to be calm—he simply was.

Years earlier, Julian had lived in constant adjustment. Fixing sleep. Managing stress. Recovering from exhaustion. Every day felt like maintenance. The nervous system reset had begun as a necessity.

Now, regulation required no attention. It functioned in the background. Julian engaged deeply with work, then disengaged fully. Emotions arose and resolved. Sleep restored him predictably. Recovery was no longer something he scheduled—it happened naturally.

Technology surrounded him, but it no longer overwhelmed him. AI tools assisted his thinking, organized his environment, and supported his rhythms. They did not compete for his attention. They respected it.

Julian realized that he was no longer optimizing himself. He was living. The nervous system reset had not turned him into something else—it had returned him to himself.

Later that day, faced with a difficult decision, Julian paused. His body did not tense. His thoughts did not race. He considered the options clearly and chose without fear. Agency felt embodied, not conceptual.

Walking outside as evening settled, Julian felt present within complexity. Life was still demanding. The world was still uncertain. But his nervous system was ready.

Nothing needed fixing anymore. There was only living, learning, and responding. The reset was complete—not as an ending, but as a beginning.

Epilogue

Living After the Reset: Sustaining Regulation in a World That Never Slows Down

The nervous system reset does not end when the final chapter is read. It begins when regulation becomes so integrated that it no longer requires conscious management. This epilogue is not a summary of techniques or concepts, but a reframing of what it means to live after recovery—when sleep restores naturally, stress resolves efficiently, awareness remains available, and the nervous system responds to life rather than bracing against it.

Modern life will not become quieter. Technology will not become slower. Demands will not disappear. The significance of the nervous system reset lies not in changing the world, but in changing how the body meets it. A regulated nervous system does not require ideal conditions. It carries stability internally. This is the difference between fragile wellness and resilient health.

After the reset, stress still appears, but it no longer accumulates silently. The nervous system recognizes activation as temporary. Recovery follows effort automatically. Sleep becomes reliable rather than negotiated. Emotional responses remain proportional and transient. These changes are subtle, but their impact compounds over time, protecting cognitive health, emotional depth, and physical vitality across decades.

One of the most important shifts after the reset is trust—trust in the body's signals, trust in recovery, and trust in one's own limits. This trust eliminates the need for constant self-monitoring. The nervous system becomes a collaborator rather than an obstacle. AI, once essential for guidance, becomes optional—present as support rather than necessity.

Living after the reset also changes how ambition is experienced. Goals no longer feel urgent in a way that threatens stability. Progress unfolds steadily rather than explosively. The nervous system allows sustained engagement without collapse. This steady trajectory often leads to greater achievement over time, even though it feels less dramatic.

Awareness remains available without effort. Presence is no longer something to practice; it is something that returns naturally whenever attention settles. This presence deepens relationships, sharpens perception, and enhances meaning without requiring withdrawal from life.

Perhaps the most profound outcome of the nervous system reset is identity transformation. Individuals stop identifying as anxious, burned out, unfocused, or overwhelmed. These states become temporary experiences rather than defining traits.

Regulation reshapes self-concept quietly but permanently.

As artificial intelligence continues to evolve, this internal stability becomes a form of protection. The regulated nervous system resists manipulation, overload, and dependency. It engages technology selectively and intentionally. This discernment preserves autonomy in an increasingly persuasive digital environment.

The epilogue does not offer a new system to follow. It offers permission to stop managing and start living. The reset has already done its work. What remains is participation—responding to life with clarity, adaptability, and trust.

The story that follows captures this final transition: not into something new, but into something sustainable. It is not a story of achievement, but of continuity—of a life lived without constant repair.

The Quiet Continuation

There was no moment when Maya declared herself healed. No milestone. No celebration. One day, she simply noticed that her life no longer revolved around recovery.

Sleep came when it was time. Stress rose and fell. Emotions moved through her without sticking. Decisions felt grounded. Her body responded to challenges without bracing for impact.

Maya remembered when every day required adjustment—monitoring energy, managing stress, fixing exhaustion. That phase had passed without ceremony.

AI still existed in her life, but it no longer led it. Tools supported her rhythms quietly. Notifications waited. Systems adapted. She remained in control without effort.

On a busy afternoon, Maya paused and felt her breath deepen naturally. No technique. No reminder. Just response. Her nervous system had learned.

Years later, friends asked how she stayed so steady. Maya struggled to answer. There was no single habit, no secret discipline. Stability had become the background rather than the goal.

Walking through a familiar street, Maya felt present. The world moved around her—noisy, fast, unpredictable—but her body remained calm within it. Not detached. Engaged.

She understood then that the nervous system reset had not changed her life externally. It had changed how life moved through her.

Nothing dramatic happened next. And that was the point.

The story continued—quietly, sustainably, fully.

www.ingramcontent.com/pod-product-compliance
Lightning Source LLC
LaVergne TN
LVHW022024200926
848481LV00007B/2532